Diabetic Smoothie, Sauce, Dip, and Dressing Cookbook

50 Easy and Healthy Diabetic Recipes for the Newly Diagnosed to Manage Prediabetes and Type 2 Diabetes

Melissa Mitchell

Table of Contents

Introduction

Diabetes Mellitus ("diabetes" for short) is a severe disease that occurs when your body has difficulty properly regulating the amount of dissolved sugar (glucose) in your bloodstream. It is unrelated to a similarly named disorder, "Diabetes Insipidus", which involves kidney-related fluid retention problems.

To understand diabetes, it is necessary first to understand the role glucose plays in the body and what can happen when glucose regulation fails. Blood sugar levels become dangerously low or high.

The tissues and cells that make up the human body are living things and require food to stay alive. The food cells eat a type of sugar called glucose. Fixed in place as they are, the body's cells are entirely dependent on the bloodstream in which they are bathed to bring glucose to them. Without access to adequate glucose, the body's cells have nothing to fuel themselves with and soon die.

Human beings eat food, not glucose. Human foods get converted into glucose as a part of the normal digestion process. Once converted, glucose enters the bloodstream, causing dissolved glucose inside the blood to rise. The bloodstream then carries the dissolved glucose to the various tissues and cells of the body.

Though glucose may be available in the blood, nearby cells cannot access that glucose without the aid of a chemical hormone called insulin. Insulin acts as a key to open the cells, allowing them to receive and utilize available glucose. Cells absorb glucose from the blood in the presence of insulin, and blood sugar levels drop as sugar leaves the blood and enters the cells. Insulin can be thought of as a bridge for glucose between the bloodstream and cells.

The body is designed to regulate and buffer the amount of glucose dissolved in the blood to maintain a steady supply to meet cell needs. The pancreas, one of your body's many organs, produces, stores, and releases insulin into the bloodstream to bring glucose levels back down.

The concentration of glucose available in the bloodstream at any given moment is dependent on the amount and type of foods that people eat. Refined carbohydrates, candy, and sweets are easy to break down into glucose. Correspondingly, blood glucose levels rise rapidly after such foods have been eaten. In contrast, blood sugars rise gradually and slowly after eating more complex, unrefined carbohydrates (oatmeal, apples, baked potatoes, etc.), which require more digestive steps to take place before glucose can be yielded. Faced with rapidly rising blood glucose concentrations, the body must react quickly by releasing large amounts of insulin at once or risk a dangerous condition called Hyperglycemia (high blood sugar) which will be described below.

The influx of insulin enables cells to utilize glucose, and glucose concentrations drop. While glucose levels can rise and fall rapidly, insulin levels change much more slowly. When a large amount of simple sugar is eaten, the bloodstream quickly becomes flooded with glucose. The pancreas releases insulin in response to the increased sugar. The glucose rapidly enters the cells, but the high insulin levels remain in the bloodstream for some time.

This can result in an overabundance of insulin in the blood, which can trigger feelings of hunger and even hypoglycemia (low blood sugar), another serious condition. When blood glucose concentrations rise more gradually, there is less need for dramatic compensation. Insulin can be released in a more controlled and safer manner, requiring the body to experience less strain. This more gradual process will leave you feeling "full" or content for a more extended period.

For these reasons, it is best for overall health to limit the amount and frequency of sweets and refined sugars in your diet. Instead, eat more complex sugars such as raw fruit, whole wheat bread and pasta, and beans. The difference between simple and complex sugars (carbohydrates) is exemplified by the difference between white (simple) and whole wheat (more difficult) bread.

Insulin is the critical key to the cell's ability to use glucose. Problems with insulin production or how insulin is recognized by the cells can easily cause the body's carefully balanced glucose metabolism system to get out of control. When either of these problems occurs, diabetes develops, blood sugar levels surge and crash, and the body risks becoming damaged.

Diabetes: Definition, Causes, And Symptoms

What Is Diabetes?

Diabetes is a disease that affects your body's ability to produce or use insulin. Insulin is a hormone. When your body turns the food you eat into energy (also called sugar or glucose), insulin is released to help transport this energy to the cells. Insulin acts as a "key." Its chemical message tells the cell to open and receive glucose. If you produce little or no insulin or are insulin resistant, too much sugar remains in your blood. Blood glucose levels are higher than average for individuals with diabetes. There are two main types of diabetes: Type 1 and Type 2.

Diabetes is a disease that occurs when your blood glucose, also called blood sugar, is too high. Blood glucose is your primary source of energy and comes from the food you eat. Insulin, a hormone made by the pancreas, helps glucose from food get into your cells to be used for energy. Sometimes your body doesn't make enough or any insulin or doesn't use insulin well. Glucose then stays in your blood and doesn't reach your cells.

What Is Type 1 Diabetes?

When you are affected with Type 1 diabetes, your pancreas does not produce insulin. Type 1 diabetes, once called juvenile diabetes, is often diagnosed in children or teens. However, it can also occur in adults. This type accounts for 5-10 percent of people with diabetes.

What Is Type 2 Diabetes?

Type 2 diabetes occurs when the body does not produce enough insulin or when the cells cannot use insulin properly, which is called insulin resistance. Type 2 diabetes is commonly called "adult-onset diabetes" since it is diagnosed later in life, generally after 45. It accounts for 90-95 percent of people with diabetes. In recent years, Type 2 diabetes has been diagnosed in younger people, including children, more frequently than in the past.

Gestational Diabetes

Gestational diabetes develops in some women when they are pregnant. Most of the time, this type of diabetes goes away after the baby is born. However, if you've had gestational diabetes, you have a greater chance of developing type 2 diabetes later in life. Sometimes diabetes diagnosed during pregnancy is type 2 diabetes.

Who Gets Diabetes? What Are The Risk Factors?

Factors that increase your risk differ depending on the type of diabetes you ultimately develop.

Risk Factors For Type 1 Diabetes Include:

- We are having a family history (parent or sibling) of type 1 diabetes.
- Injury to the pancreas (such as by infection, tumor, surgery, or accident).
- Presence of autoantibodies (antibodies that mistakenly attack your own body's tissues or organs).
- Physical stress (such as surgery or illness).
- Exposure to illnesses caused by viruses.

Risk Factors For Prediabetes And Type 2 Diabetes Include:

- Family history (parent or sibling) of prediabetes or type 2 diabetes.
- I am African-American, Hispanic, Native American, Asian-American race, or Pacific Islander.
- It is overweight.
- I had high blood pressure.
- I am having low HDL cholesterol (the "good" cholesterol) and a high triglyceride level.
- She was physically inactive.
- They were being aged 45 or older.

- I am having gestational diabetes or giving birth to a baby weighing more than 9 pounds.
- I have polycystic ovary syndrome.
- I was having a history of heart disease or stroke.
- She is a smoker.

Risk Factors For Gestational Diabetes Include:

- Family history (parent or sibling) of prediabetes or type 2 diabetes.
- Being African-American, Hispanic, Native American, or Asian-American.
- You are overweight before your pregnancy.
- They are over 25 years of age.

Symptoms And Causes

What Causes Diabetes?

The cause of diabetes, regardless of the type, is having too much glucose circulating in your bloodstream. However, the reason why your blood glucose levels are high differs depending on the type of diabetes.

1. Causes Of Type 1 Diabetes: This is an immune system disease. Your body attacks and destroys insulin-producing cells in your pancreas. Without insulin to allow glucose to enter your cells, glucose builds up in your bloodstream. Genes may also play a role in some patients. Also, a virus may trigger an immune system attack.

2. Cause Of Type 2 Diabetes And Prediabetes: Your body's cells don't allow insulin to work as it should to let glucose into its cells. Your body's cells have become resistant to insulin. Your pancreas can't keep up and make enough insulin to overcome this resistance. Glucose levels rise in your bloodstream.

3. Gestational Diabetes: Hormones produced by the placenta during pregnancy make your body's cells more resistant to insulin. Your pancreas can't make enough insulin to overcome this resistance. Too much glucose remains in your bloodstream.

What Causes Diabetes?

Genetics, lifestyle, and environment can be causes of diabetes. Eating an unhealthy diet, being overweight or obese, and not exercising enough may play a role in developing diabetes, particularly Type 2 diabetes. An autoimmune response causes type 1 diabetes. The body's immune system attacks and destroys the insulin-producing beta cells in the pancreas.

How Does Diabetes Affect My Body?

Over time, high blood sugar levels (also called hyperglycemia) can lead to kidney disease, heart disease, and blindness. The excess sugar in the bloodstream can damage the tiny blood vessels in your eyes and kidneys and can harden or narrow your arteries.

What Are The Symptoms Of Diabetes?

- Extreme thirst
- Frequent urination
- Blurry vision
- Extreme hunger
- Increased tiredness
- Unusual weight loss

What Health Problems Can People With Diabetes Develop?

Over time, high blood glucose leads to problems such as:

- Heart disease
- Stroke
- Kidney disease
- Eye problems
- Dental disease
- Nerve damage
- Foot problems

You can take steps to lower your chances of developing these diabetes-related health problems.

How Can I Find Out If I Have Diabetes?

Sometimes a routine exam by an eye doctor or foot doctor will reveal diabetes. Diabetes affects the circulation to your feet and the tiny blood vessels in your eyes. If your eye doctor or your foot doctor suspects you have diabetes, they will recommend seeing your regular physician for a blood sugar level test. The most common test is a fasting blood glucose test. After not eating for at least eight hours, your doctor will usually take a blood sample overnight. The standard, non-diabetic range for fasting blood glucose is 70 to 110 mg/dl. If your level is 126 mg/dl or greater, you may have diabetes.

How Is Diabetes Managed?

Diabetes affects your whole body. To best manage diabetes, you'll need to take steps to keep your risk factors under control and within the normal range, including:

- Keep your blood glucose levels as near to normal as possible by following a diet plan, taking prescribed medication, and increasing your activity level.
- Maintain your blood cholesterol (HDL and LDL levels) and triglyceride levels near the normal ranges as possible.
- Control your blood pressure. Your blood pressure should not be over 140/90 mmHg.

You hold the keys to managing your diabetes by:

We are planning what you eat and following a healthy meal plan. Follow a Mediterranean diet (vegetables, whole grains, beans, fruits, healthy fats, low sugar) or Dash diet. These diets are high in nutrition and fiber and low in fats and calories. See a registered dietitian for help understanding nutrition and meal planning.

- I am exercising regularly. Try to exercise for at least 30 minutes most days of the week. Walk, swim or find some activity you enjoy.
- You are losing weight if you are overweight. Work with your healthcare team to develop a weight-loss plan.
- Taking medication and insulin, if prescribed, and closely following recommendations on how and when to take it.
- We are monitoring your blood glucose and blood pressure levels at home.
- You are keeping your appointments with your healthcare providers and having laboratory tests completed as ordered by your doctor.
- I am quitting smoking (if you smoke).
- You have a lot of control – on a day-to-day basis – in

Smoothie Recipes

1. Kiwi Vanilla Yogurt Smoothie

Prep Time: 5 mins

Total Time: 5 mins

Ingredients

- 8 fl. oz. (237 ml) Glucerna Shake, Homemade Vanilla flavor
- 6 oz. low-fat Greek yogurt
- 1 medium kiwi fruit, sliced
- 4 ice cubes

Instructions

- Combine the Glucerna Shake (Homemade Vanilla), Greek yogurt, kiwi fruit, and ice cubes in a high-speed blender.
- Process for 20 seconds or until smooth.
- Pour in serving glasses.
- Serve and enjoy.

Nutrition Information

- Fat: 5.2g| Saturated fat: 1.4g| Carbohydrates: 18.6g| Sugar: 12.4g| Sodium: 221mg| Fiber: 2.6g| Protein: 12.8g| Cholesterol: 10mg

2. Dragon Fruit Smoothie Bowl

Prep Time: 3 Mins

Cook Time: 2 Mins

Total Time: 5 Minutes

Ingredients

- 3/4 cup frozen fruit (we used dragon fruit, mangoes, strawberries, and peaches)
- 1 cup spinach
- 1/2 cup Greek yogurt
- 1/2 Avocado

Instructions

- Add ingredients to blender or food processor.
- Blend on high until smooth. As needed, pause and scrape the edges with a spoon or spatula to incorporate all ingredients.
- Enjoy!

Nutritional Facts

- Carbs: 295g| Fiber: 8g| Net Carbs: 21g| Protein: 15g

3. The Ultimate Green Smoothie Recipe

Prep Time: 5 minutes

Ingredients

- 35g (1 cup, firmly packed) baby spinach leaves
- 1 Lebanese cucumber, chopped
- 1 green apple, unpeeled, cored, chopped
- 250ml (1 cup) coconut water
- ½ cup ice cubes

Method

- Put all ingredients in a blender. Cover and blend until smooth.
- Pour smoothie between 2 glasses and serve immediately.

Nutritional Value

- Protein: 2g| Total Fat: 0.3g| Satfat: 0.1g| Carbs: 16g| Fiber: 3g| Sodium: 38mg.

4. Peach Smoothie (Diabetic)

Prep Time: 10m

Ready In: 10 minutes

Ingredients

- 2 cups fat-free soy beverage (no-fat 500ml)
- 2 medium bananas (400g, chopped coarsely)
- 4 medium peaches (600g, chopped coarsely)
- 1/2 teaspoon ground cinnamon

Step 1

- Blend or process ingredients, in batches, until smooth.

Nutritional Facts

- Total Fat: 0.6g| Saturated Fat: 0.1g| Sodium: 2.9mg| Total Carbohydrate: 34.7g| Dietary Fiber: 4g| Sugars: 19.9g| Protein: 5.2 g| Calcium: 34.8mg| Iron: 2mg| Vitamin C: 15mg|

5. Diabetes-Friendly Chocolate Chia Smoothie Recipe

Total Time: 10 min Prep Time: 5 min Cook Time: 5 min

Ingredients

- ½ cup unsweetened almond milk
- 2 tablespoons chia seeds
- ½ teaspoon cinnamon
- 1 ½ medium frozen bananas, cut into chunks
- 1 ½ cups unsweetened almond milk
- 2 tablespoons cocoa powder
- 2 tablespoons peanut butter powder

Preparation

- In a medium bowl, whisk together almond milk, chia seeds, and cinnamon. Let sit for at least 10 minutes for the chia seeds to swell and absorb the liquid.
- Combine the banana, almond milk, cocoa powder, and peanut butter powder in a blender. Puree until well combined.
- Divide the chia pudding between two glasses. Top with the smoothie and serve immediately.

Nutrition Value

- Fat: 8g| Carbs: 31g| Protein: 6g

6. Lower Carb Strawberry Smoothie

Cook Time: 5 minutes

Total Time: 5 minutes

Ingredients

- 5 medium strawberry
- 1 cup unsweetened soy milk (or unsweetened almond milk)
- 1/2 cup low-fat Greek-style yogurt
- 6 ice cubes

Instructions

- Place all ingredients in a blender and blend until smooth.
- Pour into a glass and garnish with a strawberry.

Nutrition Facts

- Fat: 6g| Saturated Fat: 1g| Polyunsaturated Fat: 0.1g| Monounsaturated Fat: 0.03g| Cholesterol: 8mg| Sodium: 161mg| Potassium: 520mg| Carbohydrates: 11g| Fiber: 2g| Sugar: 6g| Protein: 16g

7. Balanced Blood Sugar Smoothie

Total Time: 10 minutes

Ingredients

- 1/2 cup Greenspring Mix
- 1/2 Banana
- 1/2 Pear, cored
- 1 1/2 cup almond milk, unsweetened
- 1 tsp rolled, gluten-free
- 1/2 tsp Cinnamon, ground

Directions

- Add ingredients in the order listed and blend until smooth.
- Enjoy!

Nutritional Information

- Total Fat: 3.9g| Saturated Fat: 0.4g| Sodium: 273.3mg|Carbs: 34.6g| Dietary Fiber: 6.2g| Sugar: 18.9g| Protein: 3g

8. Spinach Smoothie (Low-Carb & Gluten-Free)

Prep Time: 5 minutes

Total Time: 5 minutes

Ingredients

- 2 tablespoons nut butter of choice
- ½ cup plain Greek yogurt
- ½ avocado (pitted)
- ¼ cup milk (or almond milk)
- 1 teaspoon vanilla extract
- 2 cups fresh spinach
- A few drops of sweetener (to taste)
- 1 cup ice

Instructions

- Add all of the ingredients except the ice to a blender.
- Blend until smooth.
- Add the ice and pulse until the ice is mostly crushed.
- Blend until the mixture is smooth and creamy.

Nutrition Facts

- Fat: 16.1g| Saturated Fat: 2.7g| Polyunsaturated Fat: 0.7g| Monounsaturated Fat: 3.5g| Cholesterol: 8.1mg| Sodium:

66.9mg| Potassium: 473.8mg| Carbohydrates: 11g| Fiber: 4.4g| Sugar: 4.8g| Protein: 11.1g| Net carbs: 6.6g

9. Pineapple Kale Smoothie

Prep Time: 5 minutes

Total Time: 5 minutes

Ingredients

- 1 cup 0% fat Greek yogurt
- 1½ cups cubed pineapple
- 3 cups baby kale
- 1 cucumber
- 2 tbsp, hemp seeds

Instructions

Put all the ingredients in a blender (I use a Nutribullet) and blend until the smoothie has an even and silky consistency. Find yourself a spot in the sun and enjoy!

Nutrition Facts

- Fat: 5.7g| Saturated Fat: 0.3g| Polyunsaturated Fat: 2.7g| Monounsaturated Fat: 0.5g| Cholesterol: 5mg| Sodium: 80mg| Potassium: 743mg| Carbohydrates: 31.6g| Fiber: 6.4g| Sugar: 19.1g| Protein: 13.8g

10. Banana-Berry Smoothie Recipe for Diabetics

Preparation Time: 5 minutes

Ingredients

- 1 cup ice cubes
- 1 medium banana (approximately 6 inches long), sliced and frozen
- 1/2 cup frozen blueberries (not thawed)
- 1 container (8 ounces) nonfat, artificially sweetened vanilla yogurt
- 1/4 cup skim milk

Directions

- Place ice cubes at the bottom of the blender and add banana slices, blueberries, yogurt, and milk. Cover and blend in pulses until smooth, stopping frequently to stir down the ice. Serve right away. Freeze leftovers in an airtight, microwave-safe container and thaw in the microwave until slushy.

Nutrition Information

- Carbohydrates: 28g| Protein: 6g| Fat: <1g| Sodium: 80mg| Fiber: 3g

11. Diabetic Breakfast Smoothie

Total Time: 15 mins

Serves: 3-4

Ingredients

- 2 cup - Oats (ready to cook)
- 2 - Oranges (peeled and deseeded)
- 1 - Banana (ripe)
- 5 cups - Skimmed milk
- Flax seeds - 25 gms
- Walnut deshelled - 1/4 cups
- 1/2 tbsp - Coffee powder
- Honey - 1/2 tbsp
- Mint leaves - 15 gms

How To Make Diabetic Breakfast Smoothie

- Soak the oats in milk for 10 minutes.
- Add orange, banana, walnuts, flax seeds, mint leaves, coffee powder, and honey. Leave some mint leaves for garnish.
- Blend all in a food processor till smooth. Do not strain.
- Serve chilled.

Nutrition Facts

- Calories: 240| Fat: 9g

12. Berry Delicious Smoothie Pack

Total Time: 4 hours

Ingredients

- ¾ cup nonfat vanilla Greek yogurt
- 1 cup frozen strawberries
- ½ cup frozen blackberries
- ¼ cup frozen raspberries
- ¼ cup frozen blueberries
- 2 cups coconut water

How To Make It

- Spoon yogurt into an ice cube tray; freeze for 3 to 4 hours.
- Pop frozen yogurt cubes out of the ice cube tray and place them into a quart-size plastic freezer bag along with berries. (Or, to make individual portions, divide the fruit and yogurt cubes evenly between five freezer bags.) Label the bag and store it in the freezer.
- When ready to serve, pour the contents of the bag into a blender, add coconut water, and blend until smooth. (If using individual-portion bags, add only enough coconut water to reach desired thickness

Nutritional Information

- Fiber: 1g| Total Fat: 0g| Protein: 3g| Total Carbohydrate: 13g

13. Tropical Paradise Green Smoothie Pack

Total Time: 10 Minutes

Ingredients

- 2 cups spinach
- 1 avocado, diced
- 1 cup frozen pineapple chunks
- 1 cup frozen mango chunks
- ½ cup ice cubes
- 1 cup water
- 1 cup apple juice

How To Make It

- Place the first five ingredients in a plastic freezer bag. (Or, to make individual portions, divide these ingredients evenly between four freezer bags.) Label the bag and store it in the freezer.
- When ready to serve, pour the contents of the bag into a blender. Add water and apple juice. Blend until smooth. (If using individual-portion bags, add only ¼ cup apple juice and ¼ cup water.)

Nutritional Information

- Fiber: 5g| Total Fat: 7g| Protein: 1g| Total Carbohydrate: 27g

14. Chocolate Peanut Butter & Banana Smoothie Pack

Total Time: 4 Hours

Ingredients

- 1 large banana, diced
- ½ cup peanut butter
- ½ cup plain Greek yogurt
- 1 cup chocolate almond milk

How To Make It

- Spoon yogurt and peanut butter into separate sections of an ice cube tray; freeze for 3 to 4 hours.
- Pop frozen yogurt and peanut butter cubes out of the ice cube tray and place them into a quart-size plastic freezer bag along with a banana. (Or, to make individual portions, divide ingredients evenly between two freezer bags.) Label the bag and store it in the freezer.
- When ready to serve, pour the contents of the bag into a blender, add chocolate almond milk, and blend until smooth. (If using an individual-portion bag, add only ½ cup chocolate almond milk.)

Nutritional Information

- Fiber: 5g| Total Fat: 18g| Protein: 14g| Total Carbohydrate: 39g

15. Low Carb Diabetic Breakfast Smoothie

Prep Time: 3 minutes

Ingredients

- 3/4 cup frozen mixed berries
- 2 scoops of protein powder
- 1/2 cup desiccated coconut
- 1 cup almond milk - or use coconut milk
- 1 Tablespoon flaxseed oil - or olive oil
- 1/4 teaspoon vanilla extract
- 1/4 teaspoon ground cinnamon
- 5-10 drops liquid stevia - optional for extra sweetness
- 1/4 cup water - if it's too thick for your liking

Instructions

- Place everything into a blender and blend until smooth.
- Pour into a glass and you're good to go.

Nutritional Value

- Total Carbs:27g| Net Carbs:15g| Fiber:12g

16. Green Smoothie

Prep Time: 5 minutes

Total Time: 5 minutes

Ingredients

- 100 grams baby spinach fresh or frozen partially defrosted
- 1 whole kiwi peeled and chopped
- ½ whole ripe avocado pitted and diced
- 200 ml tinned coconut milk (or almond, soy, or lalacto free milk)
- ½ whole lime the juice of
- 1 tbsp flaxseed milled or ground
- Ice cubes to the consistency liked
- Sugar-free syrup optional to taste

Instructions

- Combine spinach, kiwi, avocado, coconut milk, and some cream from the top of the tin, lime, and milled flaxseed in a blender
- Add the desired amount of ice cubes and blitz to create a texture and consistency you like
- Add sugar-free syrup or sweetener to sweeten to your taste

Nutrition Value

- Carbohydrates: 12g | Protein: 9g | Fat: 47g | of which saturates: 38g | Fibre: 5g | of which sugars: 1g

17. Ayurvedic Digestive Tea

Total Time: 10 Minutes

Ingredients

- 1/2 teaspoon whole cumin seed
- 1/2 teaspoon whole coriander seed
- 1/2 teaspoon fennel seed
- 1/2 teaspoon dried rose petals

Directions

- Place all the ingredients in an 8- to 10-ounce cup.
- Heat water on the stovetop and pour over the spices.
- Steep spices and rose petals for about 5 minutes.
- Sip while it is warm. You may strain out the spices if you prefer but this is not required.

Nutritional Value

- Carbohydrates: 11g| Protein: 1g| Fat: 1g| Saturated Fat: 1g| Sodium: 14mg| Fiber: 1g

18. Spiced Citrus Tea

Total Time: 10 Minutes

Ingredients

- 1 Spiced Citrus Teabag
- Boiling water
- 1 to 2 teaspoons orange juice
- Honey (optional)
- Orange slices (optional)

Directions

- Place tea bag in cup or mug. Pour boiling water over tea bag; steep 3 to 5 minutes. Remove tea bag, pressing out liquid. Discard tea bag. Serve with orange juice and honey, if desired. Garnish with orange slices.

Nutrition Information

- Sodium: 2.5 mg

19. Tropical Green Shake

Total Time: 10 Minutes

Ingredients

- 1 cup ice cubes
- 1 cup packed stemmed kale
- 1 cup frozen tropical fruit mix
- 1/2 cup reduced-sugar orange juice beverage
- 2 tablespoons honey or agave nectar

Directions

- Combine ice, kale, tropical fruit mix, orange juice, and honey in a blender; blend until smooth.
- Pour into two glasses.

Nutrition Information

- Carbohydrates: 32g| Protein: 2g| Sodium: 20mg| Fiber: 1g

20. Honeydew Agua Fresca

Total Time: 10-20 Minutes

Ingredients

- 1/4 large honeydew melon, rind removed and cubed
- 1/4 cup fresh mint leaves
- 1/4 cup fresh lime juice (juice of 2 limes)
- 2 tablespoons sugar
- 1 1/2 cups club soda, chilled
- 4 lime wedges
- 4 mint sprigs

Directions

- Combine melon, mint leaves, lime juice, and sugar in blender; blend until smooth. (Mixture may be blended in advance and chilled for several hours.)
- Pour into a 4-cup measuring cup and stir in enough club soda to measure 4 cups.
- Pour into four glasses. Garnish with lime wedges and mint sprigs. Serve immediately.

Nutrition Information

- Carbohydrates: 24g| Protein: 1g| Sodium: 51mg| Fiber: 2g

21. Mint-Green Tea Coolers

Total Time: 10 Minutes

Ingredients

- 2 bags of green tea
- 4 thin slices of fresh ginger (about 1 inch)
- 7 or 8 large fresh mint leaves, roughly torn
- 2 cups boiling water
- 2 cups crushed ice

Directions

- Place tea bags, ginger, and mint leave in a teapot or 2-cup heatproof measuring cup. Add boiling water; steep for 4 minutes. Remove tea bags, ginger, and mint leaves; discard. Cool tea to room temperature.
- Pour 1 cup crushed ice into each of the two tall glasses. Divide tea between glasses.

Nutrition Information

- Carbohydrates: 1g| Protein: 1g| Fat: 1g| Saturated Fat: 1g| Sodium: 1mg| Fiber: 1g

22. Banana-Berry Smoothie Recipe For Diabetics

Total Time: 10 minutes

Ingredients

- 1 cup ice cubes
- 1 medium banana (approximately 6 inches long), sliced and frozen
- 1/2 cup frozen blueberries (not thawed)
- 1 container (8 ounces) nonfat, artificially sweetened vanilla yogurt
- 1/4 cup skim milk

Directions

- Place ice cubes at the bottom of the blender and add banana slices, blueberries, yogurt, and milk. Cover and blend in pulses until smooth, stopping frequently to stir down the ice. Serve right away. Freeze leftovers in an airtight, microwave-safe container and thaw in the microwave until slushy.

Nutrition Information

- Carbohydrates: 28g| Protein: 6g| Fat: <1g| Sodium: 80mg| Fiber: 3g

23. Simple Spiced Tea Mix For Diabetics

Preparation Time: 5 minutes

Ingredients

- 2 cups artificially sweetened instant iced tea mix with lemon
- 2 tubs (0.5 ounces each) powdered sugar-free orange breakfast drink mix (such as Tang)
- 1 tub (0.5 ounces) powdered sugar-free lemon-lime drink mix (such as Crystal Light)
- 1 tablespoon cinnamon
- 1 1/2 teaspoons ground cloves

Directions

- Combine all ingredients in a bowl and mix well. Store in an airtight container. To serve, put 1 1/2 teaspoons tea mix into a mug and add 8 ounces hot water. Stir well.

Nutrition Information

- Carbohydrates: 1g| Protein: <1g| Sodium: 11mg

24. Blackberry Lemonade

Preparation Time: 10 Minutes

Ingredients

- 3 cups fresh blackberries (or thawed unsweetened frozen blackberries)
- 3 cups plus 4 cups cold water
- 6 packets NutraSweet (may add more or useless depending on sweetness of blackberries)
- 1 tub (approximately 1/2 ounce) sugar-free pink lemonade mix
- 9 sprigs of fresh mint

Directions

- Place blackberries, 3 cups of water, NutraSweet, and drink mix in a blender, cover, and process until smooth. Pour half of the fruit mixture through a fine wire-mesh strainer into a 2-quart pitcher. Use a large spoon to help force juice through the strainer. Discard solids in the strainer and rinse out. Strain remaining fruit mixture. Add 4 cups of water to blackberry lemonade in a pitcher. Stir well. Serve over ice and garnish each glass with a fresh mint sprig.

Nutrition Information

- Carbohydrates: 4g| Protein: 1g| Fat: 1g

25. Banana Raspberry Refresher

Preparation Time: 2 Minutes

Ingredients

- 4 ounces nonfat, artificially sweetened raspberry cultured yogurt
- 1/2 ripe banana, cut into chunks
- 1/4 cup skim milk
- 1/2 cup ice cubes (approximately 5 cubes)

Directions

- Place all ingredients in a blender. Cover, and process until smooth and frothy. Serve immediately.

Nutrition Information

- Carbohydrates: 34g| Protein: 7g| Fat: 1g| Saturated Fat: 1g| Sodium: 85mg| Fiber: 3g

26. Chocolate Hazelnut Coffee

Preparation Time: 10 Minutes (To Brew Coffee)

Ingredients

- 6 ounces hot coffee
- 1 tablespoon chocolate hazelnut spread, such as Nutella
- 1 packet artificial sweetener
- 1 tablespoon skim milk

Directions

- Stir all ingredients together in a mug and serve.

Nutrition Information

- Carbohydrates: 10g| Protein: 1g| Fat: 5g| Saturated Fat: 1g| Sodium: 13mg| Fiber: 1g

27. Cantaloupe Cooler

Preparation time: 5 minutes

Ingredients

- 1 cup cubed cantaloupe
- 1/2 cup nonfat, no-sugar-added vanilla yogurt
- 1/4 teaspoon lemon juice
- 1 packet NutraSweet
- Dash cinnamon

Directions

- Combine all ingredients in a blender and blend until smooth.

Nutrition Information

- Carbohydrates: 20g| Protein: 6g| Fat: <1g|Sodium: 128mg| Fiber: 2g

28. Tofu Berry Smoothie

Preparation Time: 10 Minutes

Ingredients

- 1 cup frozen raspberries
- 1 cup fresh strawberries, cut into bite-size pieces
- 1/2 cup soy milk, unsweetened (shake before pouring)
- 1/3 pound (5 1/2 ounces) soft tofu, cut into bite-size pieces
- 1 cup ice
- 1/2 cup light whipped topping
- 4 tablespoons Splenda or other artificial sweeteners
- 1 teaspoon vanilla extract
- 1 teaspoon lemon juice

Directions

- Place all ingredients in a blender. Puree until smooth. Serve immediately.

Nutrition Information

- Carbohydrates: 10g| Protein: 6g| Fat: 3g| Saturated Fat: 1g| Sodium: 10mg| Fiber: 4g| Soy Protein: 5g

29. Orange Spice Coffee Mix

Preparation Time: 5 Minutes

Brewing Time: 5 Minutes.

Ingredients

- 1/2 pound freshly ground coffee
- 1/2 cup dried orange peel (can be found in the spice section of the grocery store)
- 4 teaspoons ground cloves
- 4 teaspoons ground cinnamon

Directions

- Place all ingredients in a large zip-top bag and shake to combine. Use 5 level tablespoons with 12 cups water (use more or less to suit taste). Brew coffee according to automatic-drip coffeemaker directions.

Nutrition Information

- Carbohydrates: 1g| Protein: <1g| Sodium: 5mg

30. Chocolate Avocado Smoothie

Prep Time: 5 minutes

Cook Time: 0 minutes

Total Time: 5 minutes

Ingredients

- 1/2 ripe avocado
- 3 tbsp. cocoa powder
- 1 cup full-fat coconut milk
- 1/2 cup water
- 1 tsp. lime juice
- Pinch mineral salt
- 6-7 drops liquid Stevia
- Fresh mint (for decoration)

Instructions

- Add all of the ingredients to a blender.
- Blend on high speed until smooth and creamy. If desired, add more liquid Stevia to taste.
- Garnish with fresh mint if desired and serve.

Nutrition Value

- Sat Fat: 23.4g| Poly unsat Fat: 0.7g| Mono unsat Fat: 4g| Sodium: 180.2mg| Potassium: 307.7mg| Carbohydrates: 12.1g| Fiber: 5.5g| Sugar: 2.4g| Protein: 2.3g

31. Chai Smoothie Bowl

Ingredients

For the chai tea

- 1 cup milk almond
- ½ tbsp black peppercorn
- 1 stick cinnamon stick
- ½ tbsp cloves whole
- ½ inch new ginger (thinly sliced)
- ½ tbsp natural cardamom pods (cracked)
- 1 tbsp loose leaf black tea
- 1 tsp star anise
- ½ cup of water

For The Smoothie

- 1 medium banana
- 1 oz unflavoured sun warrior protein powder
- For the topping
- ½ moderate banana (thinly sliced)
- 1 tablespoon dried goji berries
- 2 tablespoons granola

Preparation

1. Add all of the INGREDIENTS concerning the chai tea to the pot and simmer regarding 10 minutes.
2. Stress the chai tea and invite it to cool off to space temperature before you place it into the fridge.
3. Use the fantastic chai tea and include it alongside the smoothie components to a blender and mix until smooth.
4. For helping add the smoothie to a bowl and sprinkle with the topping, enjoy!

Nutrition

Calories: 410

Protein: 32g

Fat: 9g

Carbs:

60g

Fiber: 9g

Sugar: 27g

32. Banana Proteins Smoothie Bowl with Hemp and Cacao

INGREDIENTS

For the smoothie bowl

- 1 cup almond milk
- 1 moderate banana (frozen optional)
- 1 cup ice
- 1 oz unflavoured sun warrior protein powder

For The Topping

- 1 tablespoon cacao powder
- 1 tablespoon dried goji berries
- 2 tablespoons granola
- 1 tbsp hemp hearts

Preparation

1. Include the smoothie bowl elements to the blender and mix until smooth.
2. Add it to the bowl and sprinkle along with the toppings, enjoy!

NUTRITION

Calories: 405

Protein: 35g

Fat: 14g

Carbs: 46g

Fiber: 8g

Sugar: 20g

33. Matcha Smoothie Bowl with Banana Milk

Ingredients

- 1 medium banana (chopped)
- 2 tablespoons dried goji berries
- 4 tbsps fresh mint (washed and stems removed)
- ½ tsp matcha green tea extract powder
- 1 persimmon fruit (chopped)
- 1 tsp sesame seeds
- 1 cup of water

Preparation

1. Add banana, ice, drinking water, matcha powder and 1 / 2 of the mint results into the blender and blend until smooth.
2. Add the smoothie in order to the bowl and sprinkle all of those other INGREDIENTS at the top, enjoy!

Nutrition

Calories: 289 Fat: 2g Protein: 5g Carbs: 69g Fiber: 12g Sugar: 41g

34. Fruit Smoothie 2 (with milk)

Prep Time: 5 minutes

Makes: 6 cups

Ingredients

- 3 cups nonfat or 1% milk
- 3 cups fruit, sliced

Directions

1. Combine milk and fruit in a blender and put the lid on tightly.
2. Blend until smooth. Serve immediately.
3. Refrigerate leftovers within 2 hours.

Nutritional Facts

Calories: 120 Total Fat: 1.5g Sodium: 65mg Carbohydrates: 24g

Sugars: 15g Protein: 5g Dietary Fiber: 2g

35. Peach And Carrot Smoothie

Prep Time: 5 minutes

Makes: 3 cups

Ingredients

- 1 medium banana, peeled fresh or frozen
- 1 cup frozen carrots
- 1 can (15 ounces) peaches, undrained

Directions

1. Combine all ingredients in a blender or food processor including the juice or syrup from the canned peaches.
2. Blend until smooth.
3. Serve immediately.
4. Refrigerate or freeze leftovers within 2 hours.

Nutritional Facts

Calories: 130 Total Fat: 0g Sodium: 50mg Carbohydrates: 31g Sugars: 25g Protein: 2g Dietary Fiber: 3g Calcium: 17mg Iron: 0mg Potassium: 301mg Vitamin D 0mcg Vitamin A: 324mcg Vitamin C: 6mg

36. Peach Yogurt Smoothie

Prep Time: 10 minutes

Makes: 3 cups

Ingredients

- 1 cup low-fat yogurt (try peach, vanilla, or lemon)
- 1/3 cup nonfat dry milk
- 1/2 banana
- 3/4 cup orange juice
- 1/2 cup frozen peaches

Directions

1. Put all ingredients into a blender.
2. Blend until smooth.
3. Refrigerate leftovers within 2 hours.

Nutritional Facts

Calories: 130 Total Fat: 1g Sodium: 160mg Carbohydrates: 23g
Sugars: 20g Protein: 8g Dietary Fiber: 1g

37. Peanut Power Smoothie

Prep Time: 10 minutes

Makes: 4 cups

Ingredients

- ¼ cup peanut butter
- 1 ¾ cups banana (or any other fresh or canned and drained fruit)
- ¼ cup nonfat dry milk powder
- 1 ½ cups cold water

Directions

1. Put all ingredients in the blender. Blend on low until smooth, and serve.
2. Refrigerate leftovers within 2 hours.

Nutritional Facts

Calories: 180 Total Fat: 8g Sodium: 115mg Carbohydrates: 22g Sugars: 13g Protein: 7g Dietary Fiber: 3g

38. Popeye Power Smoothie

Prep Time: 10 minutes

Makes: 4 cups

Ingredients

- 1 cup of orange juice
- ½ cup pineapple juice
- ½ cup low-fat plain or vanilla yogurt
- 1 banana, peeled and sliced
- 2 cups fresh spinach leaves
- 2 cups crushed ice

Directions

1. Combine all ingredients in a blender.
2. Puree until completely smooth.
3. Serve immediately.
4. Refrigerate leftovers within 2 hours.

Nutritional Facts

Calories: 90 Total Fat: 0.5g Sodium: 35mg Carbohydrates: 20g
Sugars: 15g Protein: 3g Calcium: 77mg Vitamin D: 0mcg Vitamin
A: 81mcg Vitamin C: 42mg Iron: 1mg Potassium: 355mg

39. Pumpkin Smoothie in Cup

Prep Time: 5 minutes

Makes: 1 cup

Ingredients

- 2/3 cup low-fat vanilla yogurt or 1 container (6 ounces)
- 1/4 cup canned pumpkin
- 2 teaspoons brown sugar
- 1/4 teaspoon cinnamon
- 1/8 teaspoon nutmeg (optional)

Directions

1. Combine all ingredients in a bowl or blender.
2. Mix until smooth and serve.
3. Refrigerate leftovers within 2 hours.

Nutritional Facts

Calories: 200 Total Fat: 2.5g Sodium: 120mg Carbohydrates: 38g Sugars: 34g Protein: 9g Dietary Fiber: 9g

40. Tropical Smoothie

Prep Time: 5 minutes

Makes: 5 cups

Ingredients

- 1 cup nonfat or 1% milk
- 2 cups pineapple chunks (fresh, frozen, or canned and drained)
- 1 banana
- 1 cup of cold water

Directions

1. Put all ingredients in a blender. Put the lid on tightly.
2. Blend until smooth.
3. Pour into cups or glasses. Serve chilled.
4. Refrigerate or freeze extra portions for a fast, healthy snack.

Nutritional Facts

Calories: 140 Total Fat: 1g Sodium: 45mg Carbohydrates: 32g Sugars: 26g Protein: 4gDietary Fiber: 3g

Sauce, Dip, and Dressing Recipes

1. Keto Ranch Dressing

Prep Time:5 minutes

Cook Time:0 minutes

Resting time:1 hour

Total Time:1 hour 5 minutes

Ingredients

- 3/4 cup mayonnaise
- 3/4 cup sour cream
- 2 tbsp. fresh parsley
- 1 tbsp. fresh dill
- 1 tbsp. fresh chives
- 2 garlic cloves
- 1/2 tsp. onion powder
- 1/2 tsp. salt
- 1/2 tsp black pepper
- 1/4 cup milk of choice
- Lemon juice (optional)

Instructions

- Wash the fresh herbs and dry them completely so the excess water won't dilute the dressing. Chop them finely.
- Mince the garlic, then use a garlic press or a fork to press it into a paste.
- Add all of the ingredients to a small mixing bowl.
- Whisk together until the ranch is smooth, creamy, and there are no lumps. Adjust to taste with salt, pepper, and lemon juice, keeping in mind that the flavors will develop in the refrigerator.
- Cover and refrigerate for at least 3 – 4 hours or overnight.

Nutrition Facts

- Fat: 16g| Saturated Fat: 5.1g| Polyunsaturated Fat: 7.4g| Monounsaturated Fat: 2.9g| Cholesterol: 6.9mg| Sodium: 242.9mg| Potassium: 87.6mg| Carbohydrates: 2.7g| Fiber: 0.3g| Sugar: 1.5g| Protein: 1.1g| Vitamin A: 12.4IU| Vitamin C: 10.4mg| Calcium: 5.9mg| Iron: 2.5mg| Net carbs: 2.4g

2. Cheesy Artichoke Dip

Cook Time: 15 Min

What You'll Need

- 2 (13.75-ounce) cans artichoke hearts in water, drained and chopped
- 1 (4-ounce) can mild diced green chilies, drained
- 6 tablespoons reduced-fat mayonnaise
- 1 1/2 cup reduced-fat finely shredded Cheddar cheese, divided

What To Do

- Preheat oven to 350 degrees F. Coat a 2-cup baking dish with cooking spray.
- In a bowl, combine all the ingredients, except 1/2-cup of cheddar cheese. Spoon into baking dish. Sprinkle with remaining cheese.
- Bake 15 minutes, or until mixture bubbles and is heated through.

Nutritional Information

- Fat: 4.2g| Saturated Fat: 1.6g|Protein: 4.4g|Sodium: 284mg|Total Carbohydrates: 4.8g| Dietary Fiber: 0.7g| Sugars: 0.9g

3. Low Carb BBQ Sauce

Prep Time: 5 mins

Cook Time: 35 mins

Total Time: 40 mins

Ingredients

- 8 ounces canned tomato sauce
- 1 Tablespoon onion powder
- ¼ teaspoon garlic powder
- 1 Tablespoon chili powder
- 2 Tablespoons Worcestershire sauce with no added sugar
- 2 Tablespoons mustard dijon or regular
- ⅛ teaspoon stevia concentrated powder or ¼ teaspoon liquid
- ¼ teaspoon monk fruit concentrated powder or ½ teaspoon liquid
- 2 teaspoons liquid smoke optional for a smokey flavor
- 1 teaspoon sea salt
- 2 Tablespoons apple cider vinegar

Instructions

- Mix all ingredients in a small saucepan.
- Bring to a boil, reduce to low, and simmer uncovered for about 30 minutes, stirring occasionally. If desired, cook

boneless skinless meat in the sauce and shred for BBQ pulled pork or chicken.

Nutrition

- Carbohydrates: 2g | Protein: 0g | Fat: 0g | Saturated Fat: 0g | Cholesterol: 0mg | Sodium: 362mg | Potassium: 107mg | Fiber: 0g | Sugar: 1g | Vitamin A: 280IU | Vitamin C: 1.8mg | Calcium: 11mg | Iron: 0.5mg

4. Fat-Free Honey Mustard Sauce

Prep Time: 5 minutes

Total Time: 5 minutes

Ingredients

- 1/4 cup honey
- 1/2 cup plain nonfat greek yogurt
- 1/4 cup dijon mustard
- 1 tablespoon yellow mustard
- 1/2 teaspoon salt
- Pepper to taste
- Juice of 1 lemon

Instructions

- Simply whisk all ingredients together and chill in the fridge for 30 minutes to an hour.
- Keep refrigerated for up to a week.

Nutrition Facts

- Sodium: 110mg| Carbohydrates: 9g| Sugar: 9g| Protein: 2g

5. Chicken Marinade For Grilling

Prep Time: 2 mins

Total Time: 2 mins

Ingredients

- ½ cup olive oil
- ¼ cup liquid aminios or soy sauce
- ¼ teaspoon stevia concentrated powder see note
- ¼ teaspoon monk fruit liquid extract see note
- 2 teaspoons Worcestershire sauce
- 2 tablespoons apple cider vinegar
- 2 teaspoons garlic powder
- 1 teaspoon ginger
- 1 teaspoon black pepper
- ¼ teaspoon chili powder

Instructions

- Whisk all ingredients together in a small bowl.
- Pour marinade over chicken in large plastic zipper bags.
- Allow chicken to marinate for at least an hour.
- Brush leftover marinade on chicken during grilling.

Nutrition

- Calories: 99 | Carbohydrates: 0.8g | Protein: 0.9g | Fat: 10.8g | Sodium: 384mg | Fiber: 0.1g

6. Homemade Pesto Sauce: Nut Free

Prep time: 5 mins

Total time: 5 mins

Ingredients

- 1-1/3 cup loosely packed basil leaves
- 4 teaspoons minced garlic
- 1/4 teaspoon salt
- 1/4 teaspoon pepper
- 2/3 cup extra virgin olive oil
- 2/3 cup grated Parmesan cheese
- Optional for those without nut allergies: 4 tablespoons pine nuts

Instructions

- Ina food processor, pulse basil, garlic, salt, pepper (add pine nuts if using) until chopped.
- Add in half the olive oil and cheese and pulse to blend, add in the rest and continue to pulse until combined.
- Makes 1 cup.
- Keep refrigerated.

Nutritional Value

- Fat: 10g| Sodium: 63mg| Protein: 2g| Cholesterol: 4mg

7. Spicy Guacamole

Prep Time: 10 minutes Total Time: 10 minutes

Ingredients

- 2 Haas avocados, ripe
- 1/4 red onion
- 1 jalapeno
- 1tblsp fresh lime juice
- Sea salt

Instructions

- Cut open the avocados, remove the pits and spoon the flesh into a bowl.
- Dice the red onion and jalapeno; roll the lime to make it easier to squeeze.
- Begin breaking down avocado pieces and smash them into desired consistency.
- Add chopped vegetables and lime juice; continue mixing and smashing.
- Finish with an extra squeeze of lime juice and sprinkle sea salt over top.

Nutritional Information

- 8g Total Carbs| 3g Net Carbs| 12g Fat| 1g Protein

8. Chopped Chicken Salad

Prep Time: 5 minutes

Cook Time: 30 minutes

Total Time: 35 minutes

Ingredients

- Baked chicken
- 2 lbs. boneless skinless chicken thighs
- Olive oil spray
- ½ tsp. pepper
- ½ tsp. garlic powder
- ½ tsp. onion powder
- ½ tsp. salt
- Salad
- 3 cups kale, chopped into bite-sized pieces
- 1 cup Brussel sprouts, chopped into bite-sized slices
- 1 cup purple cabbage, sliced
- 1 carrot, cut in ribbons with a mandolin (or sliced thinly)
- 1 red onion, sliced thinly
- 1 small stalk of fennel, sliced thinly (divided)
- ¼ cup pomegranate seeds
- 1 cucumber, chopped into bite-sized pieces
- 1 tomato, diced

- ¼ cup crumbled feta (optional)
- Garlic Citrus Vinaigrette
- ¼ cup extra virgin olive oil
- 1 ½ lemon, juiced (approximately 4 tbsp. juice)
- ½ tsp. salt
- ½ tsp. pepper
- 1 garlic cloves, minced
- 1 tsp. minced fennel

Instructions

- Preheat oven to 375°F (190°C). Spray a small pan with olive oil spray and spread seasonings on both sides of chicken thighs.
- Place in pan and bake for 30 minutes or until the thickest part of the thigh reads 165 degrees. Set aside and allow to cool.
- While the chicken is baking, prepare the salad ingredients. Chop the kale, Brussels sprouts, and cucumber. Thinly slice the purple cabbage, carrot, red onion, and fennel. Dice the tomato. Toss the ingredients into a large bowl, then place them in the refrigerator until needed.
- Combine all vinaigrette ingredients in a mason jar and shake vigorously. Place in the refrigerator until needed.
- Once the chicken has cooled, chop it into bite-sized pieces and place it over the salad. Drizzle on vinaigrette and toss.

Nutrition Facts

- Fat: 16.6g| Saturated Fat: 3.7g| Polyunsaturated Fat: 1.5g| Monounsaturated Fat: 6.7g| Cholesterol 105mg| Sodium 415.3mg| Potassium: 675.8mg| Carbohydrates 14.7g| Fiber 3.8g| Sugar 5.2g| Protein 30.6g

9. Mediterranean Roasted Pepper Dip

Prep Time: 5 Min

What You'll Need

- 1 (7-ounce) jar roasted red peppers, drained and patted dry
- 1 (15-ounce) can chickpeas, rinsed and drained
- 1 (16-ounce) non-fat Greek yogurt
- 2 tablespoons chopped fresh basil
- 1 garlic clove
- 1/8 teaspoon black pepper

What to Do

- Place all the ingredients in a blender jar and process until thoroughly blended. Serve immediately, or store in the refrigerator in an airtight container until ready to use.

Nutritional Information

- Fat: 0.5g|Saturated Fat: 0.1g|Protein: 4.3g| Sodium: 111mg|Total Carbohydrates: 5.7g| Dietary Fiber: 1.2g| Sugars: 1.2g

10. Tangy Spinach Dip

Chill Time: 2 Hr

What You'll Need

- 1 (10-ounce) package frozen chopped spinach, thawed and drained
- 1/3 cup finely chopped green onions
- 1 tablespoon lemon juice
- 1 (8-ounce) container reduced-fat sour cream
- cayenne pepper
- 1/2 teaspoon garlic powder

What To Do

- Squeeze spinach between paper towels to completely remove excess moisture.
- Place all ingredients in a food processor or blender and process until smooth.
- Cover and refrigerate at least 2 hours before serving.

Nutritional Information

- Fat: 2.8g| Saturated Fat: 1.7g| Protein: 2.3g| Cholesterol: 6.6mg| Sodium: 31mg| Total Carbohydrates2.7g| Dietary Fiber: 0.8g| Sugars: 0.3g

11. South-Of-The-Border Bean Dip

Cook Time: 10 Min

What You'll Need

- 2 (15-1/2-ounce) cans pinto beans, rinsed and drained, divided
- 1 cup salsa, divided
- 1 teaspoon canola oil
- 1 onion, finely chopped
- 1 green bell pepper, finely chopped
- 3 cloves garlic, minced
- 1 tablespoon dried cilantro
- 2 teaspoons ground cumin
- 3/4 teaspoon salt
- 1/2 cup (2 ounces) shredded Cheddar cheese
- 1 tomato, chopped

What to Do

- In a blender or food processor, combine 1 can of beans and 1/4 cup salsa; blend or process until smooth.
- In a large nonstick skillet, heat the oil over medium heat and sauté the onion, bell pepper, and garlic for 5 to 7 minutes, or until tender. Add the bean mixture, cilantro, cumin, salt, and the remaining can of beans and 3/4 cup

salsa; mix well. Bring to a boil, reduce the heat to low, and simmer for 5 minutes, stirring frequently.

- Pour the mixture into a shallow serving dish, top with Cheddar cheese and tomato, and serve warm.

Nutritional Information

- Fat: 1.8g| Saturated Fat: 0.9g| Protein: 4.6g| Cholesterol: 4.2mg| Sodium: 393mg| Total Carbohydrates: 11g| Dietary Fiber: 3.1g| Sugars: 1.6g

12. Parmesan Spinach Dip

Cook Time: 30 Min

What You'll Need

- 2 (10-ounce) packages frozen chopped spinach, thawed and squeezed dry
- 1 (8-ounce) package reduced-fat cream cheese, softened
- 1/2 cup freshly grated Parmesan cheese (1 tablespoon reserved for topping)
- 1/3 cup fat-free mayonnaise
- 2 tablespoons fresh lemon juice
- 1 teaspoon garlic powder
- 1 (8-ounce) can sliced water chestnuts, drained and chopped

What To Do

- Preheat oven to 350 degrees F. Coat a 2-quart casserole dish or 9-inch pie plate with cooking spray.
- In a medium bowl, beat spinach, cream cheese, all but the reserved 1 tablespoon Parmesan cheese, mayonnaise, lemon juice, and garlic powder until well blended. Stir in water chestnuts then spoon mixture into prepared pie plate. Sprinkle with reserved 1 tablespoon Parmesan cheese then cover with aluminum foil.

- Bake 15 minutes; remove foil and cook an additional 15 to 20 minutes, or until heated through. Serve immediately.

Nutritional

- Total Fat: 3.9g| Saturated Fat: 2.1g| Protein: 4.3g| Cholesterol: 12mg| Sodium: 207mg| Total Carbohydrates: 6.2g| Dietary Fiber: 1.7g| Sugars: 2.1g

13. Italian-Style Caponata

Cook Time: 30 Min

What You'll Need

- 2 tablespoons vegetable oil
- 1 large unpeeled eggplant (about 1-1/2 pounds), coarsely chopped
- 1 medium onion, chopped
- 2 tablespoons garlic powder
- 1/2 cup chopped pimiento-stuffed green olives
- 3 ribs celery, chopped
- 1 (8-ounce) can tomato sauce
- 1/4 cup white vinegar
- 1/3 cup packed light brown sugar
- 2 dashes of hot pepper sauce (optional)

What To Do

- In a large saucepan, heat the oil over medium-high heat. Add the eggplant, onion, and garlic powder and sauté for about 5 minutes, or until the eggplant begins to soften, stirring occasionally.
- Stir in the remaining ingredients and cook over medium-low heat for 25 minutes to allow the flavors to marry.

- Serve immediately or allow to cool, then cover and chill until ready to serve.

Nutritional Information

- Fat: 2.2g| Saturated Fat: 0.3g| Protein: 0.8g| Sodium: 116mg| Total Carbohydrates: 8.7g| Dietary Fiber: 1.7g| Sugars: 6.2g

14. Springtime Dip

PREP Time: 5 Min

What You'll Need

- 1 cup fat-free Greek yogurt
- 1/2 cup low-fat buttermilk
- 1 teaspoon fresh lemon juice
- 1 tablespoon chopped fresh dill
- 1/2 teaspoon garlic powder
- 1/4 teaspoon black pepper
- 1/2 teaspoon grated lemon peel

What To Do

- In a small bowl, whisk together all the ingredients until well combined. Serve, or cover, and chill until ready to serve.

Nutritional

- Total Fat: 0.2g| Saturated Fat: 0.1g| Protein: 5.0g| Cholesterol: 0.8mg| Sodium: 37mg| Total Carbohydrates: 3.0g| Dietary Fiber: 0.1g| Sugars: 2.7g

15. Cheesy Party Bake

Cook Time: 20 Min

What You'll Need

- 1/2 cup reduced-fat mayonnaise
- 2 cups shredded reduced-fat Swiss cheese
- 1 teaspoon garlic powder
- 1 scallion, sliced thin
- Paprika for sprinkling

What To Do

- Preheat oven to 350 degrees F.
- In a bowl, combine all ingredients except paprika.
- Spoon into a 1-quart baking dish, sprinkle with paprika and bake 20 to 25 minutes or until golden and cheese is melted.

Nutritional Information

- Fat: 3.2g| Saturated Fat: 0.8g| Protein: 4.0g| Cholesterol: 7.4mg| Sodium: 86mg| Total Carbohydrates: 1.3g| Sugars: 0.5g

16. Cranberry-Nut Spread

Chill Time: 30 Min

What You'll Need

- 1 (8-ounce) package reduced-fat cream cheese, softened
- 1/2 cup sweetened dried cranberries
- 2 teaspoons finely grated orange peel
- 1/4 cup chopped toasted walnuts

What To Do

- In a medium bowl, combine all ingredients and mix well. Refrigerate 30 minutes, or until ready to serve. Serve with celery or thin wholegrain crackers.

Nutritional Information

- Fat: 3.4g| Saturated Fat: 1.4g| Protein: 1.4g| Cholesterol: 7.7mg| Sodium: 67mg|Total Carbohydrates: 4.6g| Dietary Fiber: 0.4g| Sugars: 3.3g

17. In-A-Wink Guacamole Dip

Prep: 10 Min

What You'll Need

- 2 ripe avocados, halved, with seeds removed
- 1 teaspoon grated onion
- 2 teaspoons lime juice
- 1/4 teaspoon garlic powder

What To Do

- Cut avocados into quarters and peel. In a medium bowl, mash avocado with a fork.
- Add remaining ingredients and mix well.
- Serve, or cover tightly, and refrigerate for 1 hour. This is best served the same day.

Nutritional

- Total Fat: 15g| Saturated Fat: 2.1g| Protein: 2.1g| Sodium: 7.2mg|Total Carbohydrates: 9.0g| Dietary Fiber: 6.8g| Sugars: 0.8g

18. Boo-tiful Bean Dip

What You'll Need

- 2 (15-ounce) no salt added pinto beans, rinsed and drained, divided
- 1 cup salsa, divided (see tip)
- 2 tablespoons chopped fresh cilantro, plus extra for garnish
- 2 teaspoons ground cumin
- 1/4 cup finely shredded reduced-fat Cheddar cheese

What To Do

- In a blender or food processor, combine 1 can of beans and 1/4 cup salsa; blend or process until smooth.
- In a medium bowl, combine bean mixture, cilantro, cumin, salt, and the remaining can of beans and 3/4 cup salsa; mix well.
- Spoon the mixture into a serving dish; sprinkle with Cheddar cheese and extra cilantro. Cover and refrigerate until ready to serve.

Nutritional Information

- Fat: 0.6g|Saturated Fat: 0.3g| Protein: 2.9g| Cholesterol: 1.1mg| Sodium: 169mg| Total Carbohydrates: 8.4g| Dietary Fiber: 2.5g| Sugars: 0.9g

19. Sun-Dried Tomato Pesto Dip

Cook Time: 25 Min

What You'll Need

- 2 (8-ounce) packages of reduced-fat cream cheese, softened
- 1/2 cup grated Parmesan cheese
- 1/3 cup light mayonnaise
- 2 tablespoons fresh lemon juice
- 1 teaspoon garlic powder
- 1/2 teaspoon onion powder
- 1/2 cup (approximately 10) sun-dried tomatoes, reconstituted and chopped (see note)
- 1/2 cup walnuts, toasted
- 1/3 cup packed fresh basil leaves
- 1 tablespoon grated Parmesan cheese

What To Do

- Preheat the oven to 350°F. Coat a 9-inch pie plate with cooking spray.
- In a medium bowl, beat the cream cheese, 1/2 cup Parmesan cheese, the mayonnaise, lemon juice, garlic powder, and onion powder until well blended.

- In a blender or food processor, combine the sun-dried tomatoes, walnuts, and basil; process until finely chopped.
- Add the tomato mixture to the cream cheese mixture; mix well then spoon into the pie plate. Sprinkle the remaining 1 tablespoon Parmesan cheese over the top.
- Bake for 25 to 30 minutes, or until heated through. Serve immediately.

Nutritional Information

- Fat: 9.1g| Saturated Fat: 3.6g| Protein: 4.4g|Cholesterol: 20mg| Sodium: 224mg| Total Carbohydrates: 4.6g| Dietary Fiber: 0.5g| Sugars: 2.7g

20. Tangy Onion Dip

Chill Time: 1 Hr

What You'll Need

- 1 package (8-ounce) reduced-fat cream cheese, softened
- 1 carton (8-ounce) fat-free sour cream
- 1/2 cup reduced-sugar ketchup or chili sauce
- 1 packet (1-ounce) dry onion soup mix
- 1 tablespoon fresh lemon juice

What To Do

- Beat cream cheese in a bowl until smooth. Stir in the remaining ingredients and mix well.
- Cover and refrigerate for at least 1 hour.

Nutritional Information

- Fat: 1.7g| Saturated Fat: 1.0g| Protein: 1.4g| Cholesterol: 7.1mg| Sodium: 239mg| Total Carbohydrates: 4.5g| Dietary Fiber: 0.2g| Sugars: 1.3g